UNDERSTANDING

MICRONEEDLING

PROCEDURES

FOR BEGINNERS

Everything You Need To Know,
Including Safety, And Post-Treatment
Care For Radiant Skin

DR. ALICIA SONYA

CONTENTS

DISCLAIMER

The information provided in this book is for educational and informational purposes only and is not intended as medical advice, diagnosis, or treatment. Always consult with a qualified healthcare professional before beginning any therapy, practice, or lifestyle change.

The author and publisher of this book make no representations or warranties regarding the accuracy, applicability, or completeness of the content presented. While every effort has been made to ensure the information provided is accurate and up-to-date, the field of health and wellness is constantly evolving, and the reader is advised to use discretion and seek professional guidance as needed.

This book contains references to individuals, products, websites, organizations, or other entities solely for informational purposes. The author and publisher do not endorse, sponsor, or affiliate with any of these references, nor do they receive any benefit from their inclusion. The mention of any names, trademarks, or products does not imply any association or endorsement.

The use of this book is solely at the reader's discretion. Neither the author nor the publisher shall be held liable for any damages, loss, or injury resulting from the use or misuse of the information contained herein.

ABOUT THIS BOOK

Understanding Microneedling Procedures For Beginners" offers an in-depth exploration of the increasingly popular skincare technique of microneedling, meticulously covering every aspect necessary to understand, prepare for, and maintain the benefits of this treatment. This guide opens with a solid foundation on what microneedling is, tracing its origins and evolution to provide readers with a historical perspective, and emphasizing its modern-day appeal. By clarifying who can benefit from microneedling and outlining the range of device options available, this book demystifies the process, showcasing microneedling as an accessible, versatile approach for a wide variety of skin goals and conditions.

A thorough explanation of how microneedling works provides essential scientific context, including how microneedling triggers collagen stimulation and affects the different layers of skin.

Readers will gain insight into the unique mechanism of various microneedling methods, from traditional dermarollers and mechanical devices to radiofrequency (RF) microneedling, each with its specific benefits and applications.

This guide also offers a comparison of microneedling to other popular skin treatments like laser therapies and chemical peels, so readers can make informed decisions about which treatments best suit their skin concerns.

Preparation is key to successful outcomes in microneedling, and this guide breaks down each critical step for readers to follow, including recommended pre-treatment skincare routines and behaviors to avoid.

This book sheds light on different needle depths and how they relate to specific skin concerns, guiding readers on how to set realistic expectations and formulate essential questions to discuss with their practitioners. These pre-treatment insights are complemented by an overview of microneedling techniques, with distinctions between professional and at-home tools and instructions on selecting the right tools to achieve personal skincare goals.

Safety is a primary focus, and readers will find a well-researched breakdown of potential risks and precautions to minimize them.

By understanding common side effects and how to mitigate them, readers can prepare for a safe experience, with practical tips on managing skin sensitivity and recognizing signs of potential adverse reactions.

This book also clarifies which individuals should avoid microneedling altogether to ensure optimal health and safety standards. The post-treatment section is equally comprehensive, covering essential do's and don'ts, advice on handling redness and discomfort, and the importance of sun protection following the procedure.

For long-term maintenance, readers will find guidance on building a post-micro needling skin care routine that includes the appropriate use of active ingredients such as retinoids and hyaluronic acid. Recommendations are included on when to resume exfoliation and how to avoid irritants, promoting skin health and hydration over time.

Common concerns and misconceptions are thoroughly addressed, dispelling myths about pain levels, needle depths, and the safety of at-home treatments. For those who may not initially see the results they expected, this guide offers insights on the potential reasons and alternatives, ensuring readers feel confident in their treatment choices.

Finally, the book covers the practical aspects of microneedling, such as costs, accessibility, and tips for selecting a qualified practitioner. Readers can make informed decisions about the financial side of microneedling, comparing at-home and professional treatment costs and finding tips for locating a practitioner who meets high standards of safety and cleanliness.

CHAPTER ONE

Introduction To Microneedling

Microneedling is a cosmetic procedure where fine needles puncture the skin to stimulate collagen production. By creating controlled micro-injuries, microneedling encourages the skin's healing process, leading to rejuvenation and smoother texture. Professionals typically use a microneedling device with tiny needles to work over the skin's surface, ensuring even distribution of the micro-injuries. The procedure can target various skin issues, including fine lines, acne scars, and enlarged pores.

The process usually starts with cleansing the face and applying a numbing cream to reduce discomfort.

After numbing, a specialized device with fine needles is rolled or stamped across the skin, creating microchannels. These channels allow skincare products to penetrate deeper, enhancing their effectiveness. Post-treatment, the skin may feel warm and sensitive, with a slight redness that generally fades within a day or two.

Microneedling can be performed by dermatologists, estheticians, or at home with proper training. However, professional sessions offer more advanced devices and controlled settings, resulting in better outcomes. Sessions typically last about 30 minutes to an hour, and results become noticeable over the following weeks as collagen production increases, gradually improving the skin's texture and tone.

What Is Microneedling?

Microneedling involves the use of tiny needles to create controlled skin punctures, stimulating the body's wound-healing response. This response encourages collagen and elastin production, which are essential for skin firmness and elasticity. As a minimally invasive treatment, microneedling offers noticeable improvements in skin texture and tone with minimal recovery time, making it popular for those looking for non-surgical skincare solutions.

The procedure is also known as Collagen Induction Therapy (CIT) and can be customized based on the skin's needs.

For example, deeper needle penetration is often used for more severe skin issues, while a gentler approach can address minor imperfections. The device's speed and depth are adjusted to ensure consistent application across the skin, providing a balanced rejuvenation effect.

Microneedling has expanded to address issues beyond the face, like stretch marks and scars on other body areas. It's versatile for multiple skin types and conditions, including aging skin, acne scars, and hyperpigmentation. With proper care and repeated sessions, microneedling can produce lasting improvements, especially when combined with appropriate skincare.

Origins And Evolution Of The Technique

Microneedling has roots in traditional skin practices but became popularized as a modern cosmetic procedure in the early 1990s. The initial concept was based on ancient acupuncture techniques, focusing on stimulating skin renewal. By the late 1990s, Dr. Desmond Fernandes, a plastic surgeon, developed the first modern microneedling device to treat scar tissue, leading to further advancements and popularity.

Initially, microneedling was performed with basic manual rollers with small needles. The technique has since evolved to include motorized devices that offer precise control over needle depth and speed, enhancing both the safety and effectiveness of treatments.

This innovation allows professionals to tailor the procedure to individual skin types and conditions, improving outcomes and comfort.

Today, microneedling is commonly paired with other treatments, such as PRP (Platelet-Rich Plasma) and topical serums, to maximize benefits. These combined approaches have helped make microneedling a widely accepted procedure for treating various skin concerns, and it is now performed in dermatology clinics worldwide as well as in-home settings with specialized devices.

Benefits Of Microneedling For Skin Health

Microneedling promotes collagen production, which plays a key role in maintaining skin firmness, elasticity, and smoothness.

The increase in collagen and elastin from microneedling helps reduce the appearance of fine lines, wrinkles, and large pores, leading to a more youthful appearance. This makes it a valuable option for those looking to prevent or reverse signs of aging without invasive surgery.

The controlled injury approach also encourages skin regeneration, which can improve scars from acne or surgery. Microneedling can reduce the depth and visibility of scars over time as new skin cells replace damaged tissue. For those dealing with hyperpigmentation or sun damage, microneedling can improve skin tone by breaking down pigmented cells, leading to a more even complexion.

Microneedling also enhances the absorption of topical products, such as serums and moisturizers, by creating tiny channels in the skin. This allows active ingredients to penetrate more deeply, making them more effective. By combining microneedling with quality skincare products, users can see faster, more noticeable results in both skin texture and radiance.

Who Can Benefit From Microneedling?

Microneedling can benefit individuals of various skin types and ages, though it is particularly popular among those looking to improve signs of aging, acne scarring, and overall skin texture. People experiencing early signs of aging, such as fine lines and mild sagging, can benefit from the collagen-boosting effects, which help maintain youthful skin quality. Additionally, younger individuals looking to prevent aging often turn to microneedling for its preventive benefits.

Those with acne scars or uneven skin texture may see improvement in the smoothness of their skin. Microneedling helps break down scar tissue, allowing new, healthier skin to emerge. People with hyperpigmentation or dark spots may also benefit as microneedling promotes cell turnover, which helps in fading spots over time, leading to a more even skin tone.

Microneedling can be suitable for many skin types, but individuals with active skin infections, such as acne or rosacea, should avoid the procedure until the condition is controlled. Those with a history of keloids or certain skin sensitivities may need to consult a dermatologist for specialized guidance. By adapting microneedling depth and session frequency, professionals can customize treatments to suit diverse skin needs safely.

Overview Of The Different Types Of Microneedling Devices

There are several types of microneedling devices available, each suited for different levels of use and skin concerns. The most common devices include derma rollers, automated microneedling pens, and professional-grade machines. Derma rollers are handheld tools with a rolling barrel of needles, commonly used for home treatments.

Although effective, they offer less control over needle depth and are better suited for light resurfacing treatments.

Automated microneedling pens, such as the Dermapen, are electric and allow for precise control of needle depth and speed, making them more suitable for addressing specific skin issues. These devices are widely used by professionals and require training to ensure even coverage and avoid skin damage. The controlled settings make them effective for treating a wider range of skin concerns, from mild to moderate scars to general rejuvenation.

Professional microneedling machines are more advanced, often used in dermatology clinics, and capable of delivering highly controlled, in-depth treatments. These machines offer additional settings, such as suction or radiofrequency (RF) technology, which can further enhance results. Professionals use these advanced devices for treating deeper scars, and severe skin issues, or performing combination treatments with PRP for maximum benefit.

CHAPTER TWO

How Microneedling Works

Microneedling, also known as collagen induction therapy, works by creating controlled micro-injuries on the skin's surface using tiny, sterilized needles. These needles puncture the skin at specific depths to create micro-channels, stimulating the body's natural healing response. This leads to increased collagen and elastin production, essential proteins that improve skin texture, elasticity, and overall appearance.

The microneedling process involves using a handheld device or roller equipped with fine needles that can be adjusted for different depths depending on the targeted skin concern. For instance, shallower needle depths may be used for fine lines and minor texture issues, while deeper penetration addresses acne scars and deeper wrinkles. A numbing cream is often applied before starting to minimize discomfort, and the procedure generally takes 30–60 minutes depending on the treatment area.

After microneedling, the skin may appear red and slightly inflamed, resembling a mild sunburn. This is a normal response, as the skin is working to repair itself. Over the following days, the microchannels close, and collagen production continues, enhancing skin texture and tone gradually. For best results, multiple sessions spaced 4–6 weeks apart are recommended, allowing time for the skin to heal and regenerate between treatments.

Science Behind The Microneedling Process

Microneedling's effectiveness comes from triggering the skin's wound-healing cascade. When the skin experiences micro-injuries, the body responds by increasing blood flow to the area, supplying vital nutrients, and releasing growth factors. This promotes fibroblast activity—cells responsible for producing collagen and elastin, two proteins crucial for skin structure and resilience.

These micro-injuries created by microneedling are shallow enough to avoid major trauma but deep enough to stimulate the dermis, where most collagen and elastin fibers are located. As the body heals these injuries, it naturally builds a new layer of collagen under the skin's surface, which helps fill in fine lines, scars, and wrinkles over time. This process is especially beneficial for addressing issues like acne scars, as the new collagen formation helps even out scarred skin.

The science behind microneedling also explains why it's suitable for various skin types and tones. Unlike treatments like lasers that may target specific pigmentation and risk hyperpigmentation in darker skin tones, microneedling doesn't rely on light energy. Instead, it triggers a natural biological response, making it a safer option for a wide range of skin concerns and complexions.

Skin Layers And Collagen Stimulation
Microneedling targets the epidermis and dermis, the top two layers of skin where most visible skin concerns and collagen fibers

reside. The epidermis, or outer layer, serves as a protective barrier, while the dermis beneath contains collagen, elastin, and blood vessels that contribute to the skin's structure and elasticity. Microneedling reaches into the dermis without fully disrupting the epidermis, stimulating the body's natural repair process in a controlled way.

As microneedles create tiny punctures, they stimulate a release of growth factors and collagen production specifically in the dermis. Collagen provides structure, while elastin gives skin flexibility and strength. By boosting collagen levels, microneedling improves skin firmness and reduces wrinkles and scars. This controlled injury approach accelerates cell turnover, helping old skin cells shed and new, healthier skin cells surface.

The key to successful microneedling lies in the gradual collagen buildup over multiple sessions, as each treatment encourages a cycle of collagen synthesis and repair. This stimulation leads to smoother, more resilient skin with each session, especially as older, damaged layers are replaced by fresher, more vibrant skin.

Types Of Microneedling: Mechanical, Dermarollers, And RF Microneedling

There are several microneedling methods: mechanical devices, dermarollers, and RF (radiofrequency) microneedling. Mechanical microneedling devices, like dermapens, use a motorized mechanism to adjust the needle depth and frequency of punctures, allowing for precision and control. This makes them popular for professional treatments as they offer more targeted results and customization for different skin concerns.

Dermarollers are handheld rollers with tiny needles that puncture the skin as they roll. While effective, they offer less precision than mechanical devices, and the rolling motion can tug at the skin, increasing the risk of irritation. Dermarollers are often used at home but may require extra care to avoid infection or skin damage. It's best to consult a professional before incorporating derma rolling into your skincare routine.

RF microneedling combines traditional microneedling with radiofrequency energy, which delivers heat to the dermis. This enhances collagen production by stimulating the skin's deeper layers, making it effective for more advanced skin issues like deep wrinkles and sagging. RF microneedling often provides more significant, longer-lasting results, though it's usually recommended for clinical settings due to its intensity.

Comparison To Other Skin Treatments (Lasers, Peels)

Microneedling differs from treatments like lasers and chemical peels in both technique and suitability for different skin types. Laser treatments use light energy to target specific pigmentation or skin layers, effectively treating scars and hyperpigmentation but with a risk of hyperpigmentation in darker skin tones.

Microneedling, on the other hand, doesn't rely on light energy, making it safe for a wider range of skin tones.

Chemical peels work by applying an acidic solution to exfoliate and remove dead skin layers, promoting a fresh layer of skin to the surface. While effective for improving skin tone and texture, peels may not penetrate deeply enough to address deep scars or wrinkles. Microneedling, in comparison, directly stimulates collagen production in deeper skin layers, providing long-term improvements for texture, scars, and wrinkles.

Microneedling's advantage over lasers and peels is its ability to stimulate natural collagen without heat or chemicals, reducing the risk of prolonged irritation or pigmentation changes.

Each treatment has its benefits, but microneedling is often chosen for its minimal downtime and ability to treat multiple skin issues across all skin types.

Expected Results And Timeline

After a microneedling session, initial redness and slight swelling are common and should subside within a day or two. Skin texture and tone may begin to improve within a week as the body initiates the healing response, but the most significant results usually appear over time as collagen builds up. It generally takes 4–6 sessions, spaced about a month apart, to see substantial improvements in skin firmness, fine lines, and overall smoothness.

Microneedling's results are gradual, with ongoing improvements in skin quality as collagen production continues between sessions. Many people notice that fine lines soften, pores look smaller, and scars diminish in appearance after a few sessions. By the third or fourth treatment, cumulative collagen production results in firmer, more youthful skin. Maintenance treatments every 6–12 months can help prolong these results.

Each microneedling session has a cumulative effect, making it ideal for people seeking gradual, natural-looking skin rejuvenation without the downtime associated with more invasive procedures.

While individual results may vary, consistent treatments generally yield impressive, lasting improvements in skin health and resilience.

CHAPTER THREE

Preparing For Your Microneedling Treatment

Preparing for microneedling begins with selecting a qualified and experienced practitioner. This treatment uses tiny needles to create controlled micro-injuries in the skin, stimulating collagen production. For best results, schedule an initial consultation to discuss your skin goals, and any concerns, and an evaluation of your skin type and health history. Your practitioner will use this information to design a treatment plan tailored to your needs.

In the days leading up to your appointment, maintain good hydration and minimize any activities that may increase skin sensitivity, such as prolonged sun exposure or harsh exfoliation. Some practitioners recommend using products containing hyaluronic acid or antioxidants to enhance the skin's resilience. Following any pre-treatment instructions carefully will help reduce any potential risks and maximize the effects of microneedling.

If you're preparing for an at-home microneedling session, ensure all your tools are sterile and that you fully understand the device's operation. Home treatments typically use shorter needles and require strict attention to hygiene to avoid irritation or infection. Confirm with a dermatologist or licensed practitioner about whether at-home microneedling is appropriate for your skin type.

Pre-Treatment Skin Care Routine

Starting a nourishing and protective skincare routine before your microneedling treatment will prime your skin and promote better results. Two weeks before treatment, focus on hydration by using gentle, hydrating cleansers and lightweight moisturizers. Avoid any new or potentially irritating products like retinoids, exfoliants, or strong acids, as these can increase skin sensitivity.

In the days leading up to your appointment, add antioxidants like Vitamin C into your routine to help the skin build resilience against the controlled trauma of microneedling. Sunscreen is essential; use a broad-spectrum SPF daily to protect your skin from UV damage.

Maintaining a simple, balanced skincare routine with these protective steps will prepare your skin well for the treatment process.

On the day of the appointment, arrive with a clean, bare face, free from any makeup, moisturizer, or sunscreen. If you're applying any numbing cream beforehand, follow the practitioner's guidance on proper application. Avoid shaving on the day of the treatment, as freshly shaved skin can be extra sensitive to microneedling.

What To Avoid Before Treatment

To ensure a smooth and effective microneedling experience, there are several things to avoid in the days and weeks leading up to your treatment.

First, refrain from using any products containing retinoids, salicylic acid, or benzoyl peroxide for at least 48 hours before treatment. These ingredients can make your skin more sensitive, increasing the risk of irritation during the procedure.

Sun exposure should also be minimized in the week leading up to treatment, as sunburned or inflamed skin can react poorly to microneedling. Avoid waxing, chemical peels, or any exfoliating treatments that might make the skin more sensitive.

If you're taking any medications that increase sun sensitivity or thin the skin, such as certain acne medications, consult with your practitioner to determine when to discontinue use before your treatment.

Alcohol, smoking, and caffeine can affect your body's ability to heal, so reducing or eliminating them a few days prior can improve your results. To lower the risk of bruising, avoid blood-thinning supplements and medications like aspirin, fish oil, and vitamin E. By following these guidelines, your skin will be in the optimal condition for microneedling, leading to better outcomes.

Understanding Different Needle Depths For Specific Skin Issues

Microneedling uses varying needle depths to target specific skin concerns effectively. Shallow depths (0.25–0.5 mm) are commonly used for mild treatments, helping to improve skin texture, promote product absorption, and give a gentle rejuvenating boost. These depths are ideal for beginners or those with sensitive skin who want a light treatment without downtime.

For treating fine lines, wrinkles, and hyperpigmentation, slightly deeper needles (0.5–1.0 mm) are typically applied. These depths penetrate further into the dermis, where collagen and elastin fibers are more active. Practitioners often use this depth for individuals looking to reduce early signs of aging or sun damage, as it reaches the layer of skin where rejuvenation processes are most effective.

Deeper treatments (1.5–2.5 mm) are generally reserved for severe scarring or stretch marks, as these target the skin's deeper layers to remodel collagen more intensively.

Only qualified professionals should perform treatments at this level due to the potential for more significant skin trauma and longer healing times. Consulting your practitioner to determine the right depth for your skin concerns ensures the best, safest results.

Questions To Ask Your Practitioner

When consulting a practitioner for microneedling, it's essential to ask questions that clarify the procedure and ensure you're in capable hands. Start by asking about their experience and training, especially with microneedling treatments. Request information about the devices they use, as different microneedling pens or rollers can vary in effectiveness, safety, and suitability for different skin types.

Another key question is about the expected results and any potential side effects. A trustworthy practitioner will provide a realistic timeline for when you can see improvements, along with details on what you might experience in terms of skin redness, tenderness, and possible mild flaking. Asking how many sessions you may need for your skin goals is also helpful, as treatments are often spaced about four to six weeks apart for optimal results.

Finally, ask about pre- and post-care instructions, as these play a crucial role in achieving the best outcomes. Your practitioner should outline steps to follow to avoid infections, minimize swelling, and improve healing.

Ensuring you have a thorough understanding of what the treatment involves will help you feel confident and prepared.

Setting Realistic Expectations

Microneedling can provide significant improvements in skin texture, firmness, and clarity, but it's essential to set realistic expectations. Initial results, such as a subtle glow and smoother skin texture, are often visible within a week of treatment. However, since the main benefits come from collagen production, which takes time, full results typically develop over the next few months with a series of treatments.

Microneedling is effective for addressing fine lines, minor scarring, and enlarged pores, but it is not a one-time fix.

Patients with deep scars or pronounced wrinkles may need several sessions before seeing substantial improvement, and even then, results may be gradual rather than instant. Keep in mind that consistent skincare between treatments also plays a major role in supporting and enhancing results.

Understanding that microneedling may require a commitment to multiple treatments and a proper skincare routine helps you stay patient and satisfied with your progress. Communicate openly with your practitioner about your goals and listen to their professional guidance on what microneedling can and cannot achieve. This approach will ensure you have a positive experience aligned with achievable skin goals.

CHAPTER FOUR

Microneedling Techniques And Tools

Microneedling is a skin treatment that involves creating tiny punctures on the skin's surface using fine needles, prompting natural healing and collagen production. This process helps reduce the appearance of scars, fine lines, and uneven skin tone. The treatment can be performed with various tools, each designed to puncture the skin at a specific depth depending on individual needs. The key to a successful microneedling session is using the right technique and applying the correct pressure to avoid skin damage while ensuring effectiveness.

There are several microneedling tools available, from simple derma rollers to advanced dermapens and radiofrequency (RF) devices. Each tool offers a different level of precision and depth control. Dermarollers, for instance, have a roller head with rows of needles, which roll across the skin. In contrast, dermapens use a pen-shaped device with adjustable needle depths, allowing for a more controlled approach. RF microneedling adds radiofrequency energy to the needle pricks, enhancing skin rejuvenation with heat.

To achieve effective results, it's essential to follow a step-by-step approach. Start by disinfecting the microneedling tool and cleaning the skin thoroughly. Using a steady, gentle hand, apply even pressure and move the tool across the skin in consistent strokes or circular motions, focusing on one area at a time. After the procedure, apply a hydrating serum to help the skin heal, as microneedling opens channels for increased absorption of skincare products.

Overview Of At-Home Vs. Professional Tools

At-home microneedling devices, like basic derma rollers and light-duty dermapens, are designed for ease of use and limited depth, usually up to 0.5 mm. They're suitable for beginners or those looking for gentle skin improvement.

Professional tools, on the other hand, reach greater depths, sometimes exceeding 2 mm, making them ideal for treating deeper scars and advanced skin issues. These professional devices are often used by dermatologists or licensed estheticians and are generally considered safer for intense treatments due to skilled handling.

At-home tools are accessible and provide some benefits, but they come with limitations. For example, at-home derma rollers can enhance product absorption and improve skin texture slightly. However, deeper issues like acne scars or pronounced wrinkles often require the precision and strength of professional tools. Additionally, licensed professionals can use advanced devices like RF microneedling machines, which aren't available for home use but deliver more intense and longer-lasting results.

Those deciding between at-home and professional microneedling should consider skin goals, comfort level, and budget. While at-home devices are affordable and provide mild skin benefits, professional treatments are more potent and effective for significant concerns. Beginners are often encouraged to start at home with gentle tools, moving to professional sessions as their skin becomes more resilient and accustomed to the process.

Dermarollers, Dermapens, And RF Microneedling Devices

Dermarollers are handheld devices with a cylindrical roller covered in tiny needles. These needles create micro-injuries as the roller is gently moved across the skin. Dermarollers are best for beginners who want an affordable, simple tool for basic skin texture improvement. They're widely available and come in different needle lengths, typically ranging from 0.2 mm to 0.5 mm for at-home use, which is ideal for superficial treatment.

Dermapens are pen-shaped devices with needle tips that move up and down rapidly to create punctures in the skin. Unlike derma rollers, derma pens allow for adjustable needle depth, providing customized treatment for different skin areas and concerns. Dermapens also offer more precision, making them suitable for targeting specific areas with deeper acne scars or fine lines, as well as reducing the risk of tearing the skin.

RF microneedling devices add radiofrequency energy to the procedure, enhancing collagen production and skin tightening through heat. This tool is typically used by professionals, as it requires training to operate safely and effectively. RF microneedling can address more advanced skin issues, such as loose skin, deep wrinkles, and severe acne scars, and offers results that last longer than traditional microneedling.

How To Choose The Right Tool For Your Skin Goals

Selecting the right microneedling tool depends largely on your skin goals and tolerance for intensity. For minor texture improvement and product absorption, a derma roller with a needle length of 0.2 to 0.5 mm is generally sufficient and safe for at-home use. However, those looking to treat more noticeable concerns, like deeper acne scars, may benefit from a derma pen that allows adjustable needle depth, enabling a more targeted approach.

If your goals include firming and rejuvenating aging skin, RF microneedling may be more appropriate. This tool combines micro-injuries with heat, helping to stimulate deeper collagen production, which is beneficial for reducing sagging and wrinkles. However, RF microneedling is best administered by a professional due to the equipment's complexity and intensity, making it safer and more effective.

Consulting with a dermatologist or skin specialist can provide additional guidance. They can assess your skin type and needs, recommending the best tool and treatment plan. Beginners are often encouraged to start with gentler, at-home tools before advancing to professional treatments, which are more intense but yield longer-lasting results.

Proper Techniques For Safe Microneedling

Start by disinfecting your microneedling tool and cleaning your skin with a gentle cleanser. Pat the skin dry, and consider using a numbing cream for comfort, especially if you're using a tool with a needle length of 0.5 mm or longer. To begin, apply light pressure and move the tool evenly over the skin, section by section, ensuring you cover the entire area without going over the same spot multiple times to avoid skin irritation.

For derma rollers, use a vertical, horizontal, and diagonal pattern across each section to ensure thorough coverage.

If using a derma pen, hold the pen at a 90-degree angle and press it gently into the skin, moving it in small circular motions or using light tapping motions, depending on the device's instructions. Avoid the eye area, and focus on high-impact zones like the forehead, cheeks, and jawline.

After microneedling, apply a soothing serum or hydrating mask to calm the skin and promote healing.

Avoid using active skincare ingredients, like retinol or exfoliants, for at least 24 hours, as these can further irritate the skin. Additionally, wear sunscreen diligently, as microneedled skin is more sensitive to UV exposure.

Frequency Of Treatments For Optimal Results

For at-home treatments, microneedling can typically be done once every two weeks if using a dermaroller with shorter needles (0.2 to 0.5 mm), allowing the skin time to heal between sessions. As the skin becomes accustomed, sessions can sometimes be increased to weekly, but it's best to monitor how your skin responds. Overusing at-home tools can lead to irritation and potential skin damage, so gradual adjustment is crucial.

Professional treatments, which reach greater depths, generally require longer recovery times, often spaced four to six weeks apart. This spacing allows the skin to fully recover and rebuild collagen between sessions.

For more intense treatments, such as RF microneedling, sessions are spaced further apart, with results often noticeable for several months afterward.

Each skin type responds differently, so adjusting frequency based on how your skin heals is essential. Keeping track of changes in texture, fine lines, and tone will help determine if sessions are needed more or less frequently. Starting slowly and increasing as needed will optimize results while minimizing the risk of irritation or injury.

CHAPTER FIVE

Safety Precautions And Risks

Microneedling is generally a safe procedure, but following strict safety precautions is essential for minimizing risks. Before starting, ensure all equipment, especially the microneedling device, is thoroughly sanitized or replaced with a new, sterile needle cartridge to prevent infections. Also, if you're new to microneedling, consider having it done by a licensed professional to get familiar with the proper techniques. Wearing gloves during the procedure can further prevent contamination.

It's vital to prep the skin carefully. Start by washing your hands and face with an antibacterial cleanser to remove oils and dirt.

After cleaning, apply a numbing cream if needed, and allow it to set for 15-20 minutes before removing it with a clean cloth. Using a hyaluronic acid serum before microneedling can help the device glide more smoothly, reducing discomfort.

After the procedure, avoid using any products that contain alcohol, retinol, or acids on your skin for at least 24-48 hours, as they can irritate. Refrain from direct sun exposure, as microneedling increases skin sensitivity. Wear sunscreen if you must go outside, and avoid wearing makeup for at least a day to allow the skin to heal.

Common Risks And Side Effects

Some common side effects of microneedling include redness, swelling, and minor skin irritation. These are typically mild and should subside within 24 to 48 hours. To ease these effects, you can apply a gentle moisturizer or a cooling gel recommended by your provider, which can help soothe the skin as it recovers.

Microneedling may also result in small pinpoint bleeding, which is normal when the skin is punctured by the needles. However, excessive bleeding may indicate that the needle depth is too high or that the technique was too aggressive. If this occurs, it's best to pause and consult a professional before continuing.

In rare cases, microneedling can trigger hyperpigmentation, scarring, or flare-ups in people with specific skin conditions like acne or rosacea.

These risks are higher if the procedure is not done correctly or if you have underlying skin sensitivities. If you notice any worsening of symptoms, it's essential to consult a dermatologist.

Minimizing Infection And Irritation Risks
Minimizing the risk of infection starts with using clean, sanitized equipment. Ensure the microneedling device is sterilized, or use a single-use needle cartridge. It's also essential to thoroughly clean the skin and apply an antiseptic before starting, as any bacteria on the skin's surface can lead to infection post-treatment.

Keeping your hands off the treated area after microneedling is crucial for minimizing irritation.

The skin is particularly vulnerable post-procedure, so avoid touching, scratching, or picking at it to prevent bacteria from entering the newly created microchannels. Use a gentle, non-comedogenic moisturizer to keep the area hydrated and reduce dryness or itchiness.

Avoid exposure to high temperatures, like steam rooms, hot showers, or saunas, for at least 48 hours post-micro needling. The increased blood flow in these settings can exacerbate irritation and prolong the healing process.

By following these steps, you can help reduce the risk of infection and keep your skin comfortable during recovery.

What To Do If You Experience Adverse Effects

If you experience swelling, redness, or discomfort beyond the usual healing period, apply a cool compress to soothe the area and reduce inflammation. You can also apply a gentle, fragrance-free moisturizer with ingredients like aloe vera or hyaluronic acid to help calm the skin. Over-the-counter anti-inflammatories, like ibuprofen, may help reduce swelling as well.

Persistent itching or burning sensations can be managed by using a calming gel or a dermatologist-recommended serum specifically designed for post-micro needling care. Avoid scrubbing or exfoliating the skin, as this can increase irritation and prolong recovery.

Refrain from using any active skincare products, such as retinoids or acids, until the skin has fully recovered.

If adverse effects do not improve within a few days or if symptoms worsen, contact a dermatologist. They may recommend a topical antibiotic if there are signs of infection or suggest a soothing treatment plan to help the skin recover safely. Seeking professional guidance early can prevent complications from worsening and ensure your skin heals smoothly.

Understanding Skin Sensitivity And Allergic Reactions

Microneedling can make the skin more sensitive, especially to products containing fragrances, alcohol, or strong actives.

Start with a patch test for any new skincare product after microneedling to check for irritation or allergic reactions. It's best to keep your skincare routine minimal post-treatment, focusing on hydration and gentle protection.

Allergic reactions can include itching, swelling, and redness that lasts beyond 48 hours. If you experience these symptoms, avoid applying any more products and rinse the area with cool water. Use a gentle, hypoallergenic moisturizer to keep the skin calm and avoid further irritation. Anti-inflammatory creams, as recommended by a dermatologist, may also help soothe an allergic reaction.

People with conditions like eczema, psoriasis, or rosacea should exercise caution, as microneedling may trigger flare-ups.

Discussing your skin's specific needs with a dermatologist before treatment can help prevent adverse reactions. If your skin is highly sensitive, consider consulting a professional to explore milder forms of microneedling or alternative treatments.

Who Should Avoid Microneedling?

Certain individuals should avoid microneedling due to skin conditions or other medical factors. Those with active acne, open wounds, or infections should not undergo microneedling, as it can worsen the condition and increase the risk of infection. Microneedling is also not recommended for individuals with a history of keloid scarring or skin conditions that affect wound healing. Pregnant or breastfeeding individuals should consult a healthcare provider before microneedling, as hormonal changes can make the skin more sensitive, potentially leading to adverse reactions. Additionally, individuals undergoing treatments like chemotherapy or with weakened immune systems should avoid microneedling until they have recovered fully.

If you're using blood-thinning medications, consult your doctor before microneedling, as these can increase the likelihood of bruising and bleeding. Similarly, those with recent laser treatments, sunburn, or recent Botox injections should wait until their skin has fully healed before proceeding. By following these guidelines, you can ensure that microneedling is safe and effective for your skin type.

CHAPTER SIX

Immediate Post-Treatment Care

After a microneedling session, the skin needs time to heal, so it's important to treat it gently. Start by rinsing your face with cool, clean water instead of using harsh cleansers. Avoid scrubbing the skin—lightly pat it dry with a soft towel to avoid irritation. Avoid applying makeup for at least 24 hours since the tiny channels created by the needles need time to close.

Your skin may feel tight, warm, or mildly sensitive, which is normal. To reduce this, apply a soothing serum or cooling gel recommended by your technician. Hydration is key; using a hyaluronic acid serum will help replenish moisture.

Stay away from heavy creams immediately after treatment to let the skin breathe.

Minimize touching your face to avoid introducing bacteria. If you have microneedling on your body, wear loose clothing to prevent rubbing against the treated areas. Let your skin repair naturally without interference—this ensures you get the best results with minimal risk of complications.

Essential Do's And Don'ts After Treatment

Apply calming, fragrance-free moisturizers to support healing. Keep yourself hydrated by drinking plenty of water throughout the day to help the skin regenerate faster. You can use a mild, pH-balanced cleanser for gentle washing after the first day.

Don't use exfoliants, alcohol-based toners, or retinol for at least a week after microneedling. These can irritate your skin or slow down the healing process. Avoid swimming, saunas, and intense exercise for 48 hours to prevent infections, as sweat and chlorine can compromise recovery.

Do be patient with your skin's healing process. It may take a few days to a week for visible improvement to appear, so avoid picking at any scabs or flakes. Keep makeup and harsh skincare to a minimum during this period to give your skin the best chance to recover.

How To Handle Redness, Swelling, And Discomfort

Redness is expected after microneedling, often resembling a sunburn. This can last for

24 to 48 hours, but using a soothing gel with aloe vera or calendula can speed relief. For swelling, apply cold compresses in 10-minute intervals, ensuring you don't press too hard.

Discomfort is usually mild but manageable. If your skin feels tight, use a hydrating serum or light moisturizer to restore comfort. Avoid taking anti-inflammatory medications like ibuprofen, as these may interfere with the body's natural healing response.

Sleeping with your head slightly elevated can also help reduce swelling overnight. Stick to your back to avoid pressing your face into pillows, which could irritate the treated areas. In cases of excessive swelling or irritation, consult your provider promptly for advice.

Importance Of Sun Protection Post-Microneedling

Post-treatment skin is more vulnerable to UV rays, so applying broad-spectrum sunscreen (SPF 30 or higher) is crucial. Use mineral sunscreens with zinc oxide or titanium dioxide to minimize irritation while providing effective protection. Reapply every two hours, especially if outdoors.

Avoid direct sun exposure for at least one week. Wearing a wide-brimmed hat and sunglasses offers extra defense, especially when going outside during peak sun hours. Sunburn during this sensitive time can cause hyperpigmentation or delay recovery.

Even after the initial healing phase, maintaining a solid sun-protection habit ensures long-term benefits from your microneedling results. Healthy, shielded skin is less prone to discoloration, dryness, and premature aging, helping you maximize your investment.

Recommended Products For Post-Treatment Skin Care

A hyaluronic acid serum is a must for replenishing moisture and supporting faster healing. Look for products free from fragrances and alcohol to avoid unnecessary irritation. Peptide serums can also promote collagen production, enhancing the overall outcome of the procedure.

Gentle cleansers that don't strip the skin's natural oils are ideal for post-micro needling care. A fragrance-free moisturizer with ceramides or glycerin will lock in hydration. Avoid heavy or comedogenic products, as they may clog pores during the healing process.

If your skin feels particularly dry or tight, facial mists with soothing ingredients like rose water can offer instant relief. Your technician might also recommend antioxidant-rich creams to protect the skin from environmental stressors. Use products approved by professionals to ensure safety and effectiveness.

Managing Dryness And Peeling

Dryness and mild peeling often occur as the skin renews itself. To manage this, apply a rich, non-comedogenic moisturizer two to three times daily. Avoid picking or peeling at flaking skin—let it shed naturally to prevent scarring or irritation.

Incorporate hydrating masks a few days after the treatment to restore moisture levels. A gentle, overnight hydrating cream can also help if dryness persists. Drinking plenty of water aids in keeping the skin supple from the inside.

If peeling becomes uncomfortable, avoid harsh exfoliators and switch to mild, hydrating products. Products with hyaluronic acid or squalane are ideal during this phase, ensuring the new skin remains soft and healthy without triggering irritation.

CHAPTER SEVEN

Long-Term Skin Care After Microneedling

After microneedling, consistent, gentle skincare is essential for long-term skin health and achieving the best results. The skin typically remains sensitive for several weeks post-treatment, so using mild, non-irritating cleansers and moisturizers is crucial. Gentle products that don't contain alcohol, fragrances, or exfoliating ingredients are ideal to avoid aggravating newly treated skin.

Opt for cleansers that cleanse without stripping away essential moisture, and apply a rich, hydrating cream to protect the skin barrier as it heals.

Sun protection becomes more critical after microneedling, as the skin is more prone to sun damage due to its sensitivity. Wearing a broad-spectrum sunscreen with SPF 30 or higher, even indoors, helps prevent hyperpigmentation and further irritation. It's recommended to apply sunscreen daily, reapplying every two hours if outside, and to avoid direct sun exposure as much as possible, especially in the first few weeks post-procedure.

Incorporating antioxidants, like vitamin C serums, into your skincare routine after a few days can support healing and protect you from environmental stressors. However, introduce them slowly and cautiously, observing for any irritation.

These antioxidants not only help soothe inflammation but also enhance collagen production, further complementing the microneedling results.

Building A Routine To Maintain Results

To maintain the benefits of microneedling, a consistent skincare routine is essential. Begin by cleansing your face with a gentle, hydrating cleanser to remove impurities without stripping the skin's natural oils. Following this, applying a toner with soothing ingredients like chamomile or rose water can help balance the skin's pH and add a layer of moisture.

Your daily routine should include a serum, particularly one containing hyaluronic acid, which will help lock in hydration and enhance the skin's plumpness.

Follow this with a lightweight, nourishing moisturizer to further seal in hydration, especially during colder months when the skin can easily dry out. You may also want to incorporate a high-quality sunscreen as the final step in your morning routine to protect your skin from harmful UV rays.

Weekly treatments, like hydrating masks, can help sustain the glowing effects of microneedling. Masks with ingredients such as aloe vera, cucumber, or ceramides offer added moisture and barrier support.

Over time, a balanced regimen like this can support skin texture and help you retain a more youthful, radiant appearance.

Using Retinoids, Hyaluronic Acid, And Other Active Ingredients

After microneedling, it's generally advised to wait around 3–7 days before reintroducing strong active ingredients like retinoids or AHAs. Start with mild concentrations and gradually build up to avoid irritating the skin. Retinoids are especially beneficial as they stimulate cell turnover and collagen production, but always apply these in the evening to avoid sun sensitivity.

Hyaluronic acid, however, is safe to use almost immediately and can be a great addition to help hydrate and plump the skin as it recovers. This ingredient attracts moisture, which aids in reducing the appearance of fine lines and gives the skin a firmer, more youthful look.

It can be layered under a moisturizer and is generally non-irritating, making it an excellent go-to post-micro needling treatment.

Other active ingredients, like vitamin C, can be incorporated gradually to help with skin brightness and even tone. It's best to start with lower concentrations (around 10–15%) and monitor the skin's reaction. Apply these ingredients in the morning to maximize antioxidant protection during the day, while using hydrating products, like hyaluronic acid, to complement them.

When To Start Using Exfoliants Again

Exfoliating the skin post-micro needling requires a cautious approach. Ideally, give your skin at least 10–14 days before reintroducing exfoliants such as AHAs, BHAs, or physical scrubs. This waiting period allows the skin to heal and minimize the risk of irritation. When starting again, opt for a gentle exfoliant, like a low-percentage glycolic or lactic acid, and use it only once per week initially.

Chemical exfoliants, like salicylic acid, can be beneficial for acne-prone skin but should also be used sparingly at first. Apply in the evening and observe any reactions closely; if any redness or irritation occurs, reduce frequency or try an even milder exfoliant. Gradual use will allow you to build up tolerance without compromising the microneedling results.

Physical scrubs should be reintroduced cautiously and only if they are very gentle.

Avoid abrasive or grainy textures that might scratch or irritate the skin. Instead, opt for smooth, non-irritating formulas and keep exfoliating sessions brief to maintain the skin's newfound resilience and smooth texture.

Avoiding Common Skin Irritants Post-Treatment

After microneedling, steer clear of potential irritants to avoid damaging the sensitive skin barrier. Harsh cleansers, fragranced products, and alcohol-based toners can inflame the skin, causing discomfort and even leading to delayed healing.

Instead, use soothing, fragrance-free products designed for sensitive skin, which will provide calming effects without irritation.

For several weeks post-treatment, avoid direct exposure to environmental pollutants like smoke or dust as these can easily penetrate your skin's temporarily enlarged pores. Try to stay in clean environments and wash your face gently after being outdoors. Wearing a hat and minimizing sun exposure, especially when UV levels are high, can help shield skin from potential environmental damage.

Makeup, particularly heavy foundation, should also be avoided for the first few days after microneedling. If you need to wear makeup, opt for a lightweight, non-comedogenic formula, but keep usage minimal. This allows the skin to breathe and prevents potential clogging of the pores, helping your skin recover faster and maintain its post-treatment glow.

Benefits Of Continued Hydration And Nourishment

Maintaining optimal hydration is crucial after microneedling, as well-hydrated skin heals faster and looks healthier. Regular use of hyaluronic acid serums, which pull water into the skin, can help maintain a plump and dewy appearance. Additionally, drink plenty of water to support hydration from within, which will further promote recovery and enhance the skin's resilience.

Nourishing ingredients like peptides, ceramides, and fatty acids can also strengthen the skin barrier, making it more resistant to future damage.

Moisturizers with these ingredients applied twice daily ensure the skin remains well-protected, while soothing redness and inflammation. Consider a weekly hydrating mask to boost moisture retention and enhance your skincare routine.

A diet rich in skin-nourishing foods, such as fruits and vegetables high in antioxidants and omega-3 fatty acids, can provide the nutrients necessary for skin repair and rejuvenation.

Over time, combining hydration, nourishment, and a balanced diet will help sustain the results of microneedling, keeping your skin looking radiant and youthful.

CHAPTER EIGHT

Common Concerns And Misconceptions

Microneedling is often met with various concerns, mainly because the idea of puncturing the skin with tiny needles can seem daunting. Many worry about the risk of infection, and scarring, and whether microneedling will help improve their skin.

To ease these worries, it's helpful to understand that microneedling is generally safe when performed by a trained professional using sterile equipment. The small punctures trigger a natural healing response that can improve skin texture, and fine lines, and even help with hyperpigmentation over time.

Another frequent misconception is that microneedling will cause permanent scarring or severe damage. In reality, the needles used are quite small, and the controlled micro-injuries typically heal quickly without permanent marks, as long as proper aftercare is followed.

Using a professional-grade serum or moisturizer recommended by your dermatologist will also help speed up recovery and avoid complications, ensuring that your skin benefits from the procedure.

Some people are also unsure about the efficacy of microneedling on different skin types and tones. Fortunately, microneedling is compatible with almost all skin types, including darker tones, since it doesn't carry the risk of hyperpigmentation often associated with certain laser treatments. Still, individuals with active acne, skin infections, or certain medical conditions should avoid microneedling to prevent adverse reactions and achieve the best results.

Addressing Pain Levels During Microneedling

Pain is one of the top concerns with microneedling, but it's often less intense than people imagine. Most professional microneedling sessions start with applying a numbing cream to the area being treated. This numbing step minimizes discomfort and allows for a more relaxed procedure. Patients typically feel only mild pressure or a light scratching sensation, which varies based on individual pain tolerance and the depth of the needle.

For those concerned about pain at home, using shorter needle lengths is advisable. While the sensation might still be noticeable, shorter needles generally cause less discomfort and are gentler on the skin. At-home devices should not exceed 0.25 mm in needle depth, as higher depths are reserved for professional use to avoid unnecessary pain and potential complications. Shorter needles can still effectively improve the skin's texture and absorption without causing substantial discomfort.

Post-procedure, some may experience mild redness and tenderness, similar to a sunburn.

Applying a soothing, hydrating serum or cream right after treatment can ease discomfort and speed up recovery. Most of these post-treatment effects resolve within a day or two, so while there may be some initial pain, it's generally manageable and short-lived.

Dispelling Myths About Needle Depth And Skin Damage

One common myth is that deeper needle penetration guarantees better results. In reality, the appropriate needle depth depends on the skin issue being targeted and individual skin sensitivity. Superficial treatments with shallow needles (0.25 to 0.5 mm) are generally sufficient for boosting skin texture and radiance, as they stimulate the production of collagen without deep tissue impact. Deeper treatments (1.0 to 2.5 mm) are only suitable for more stubborn scars or wrinkles and should be done by trained professionals.

Another misconception is that microneedling can permanently damage the skin's surface. When performed correctly, microneedling creates tiny channels that trigger a healing response, which can strengthen and rejuvenate the skin. However, improper technique or using needles that are too deep can risk irritation, scarring, or pigmentation issues, particularly for sensitive skin types.

It's essential to follow proper guidelines and seek professional advice to determine the appropriate depth for your goals.

Professionals assess skin type, condition, and treatment goals to select the right depth and technique, so deeper is not necessarily better. With the correct approach, microneedling provides a balanced solution to skin issues without risking unnecessary harm.

Is At-Home Microneedling Safe?

At-home microneedling can be safe and effective when done carefully with the right tools and techniques. However, it's essential to use shorter needles—ideally 0.25 mm or shorter—to avoid excessive irritation and skin damage.

Shorter needles minimize the risk of infections and are primarily used to boost product absorption and enhance skin texture, making them suitable for home use. Always start with clean skin and disinfect the roller before and after each use to maintain hygiene.

While it's possible to achieve noticeable improvements at home, it's essential to avoid pressing too hard. Pressing lightly and moving the roller in small, consistent sections across the skin helps prevent irritation. Additionally, combining microneedling with a quality serum designed for post-treatment can optimize results without risking irritation. Use only serums that are safe for post-micro needling, avoiding any harsh or active ingredients.

At-home treatments may not be as intense as professional ones, but they can still yield smoother, brighter skin over time. If done correctly and patiently, at-home microneedling can be a valuable part of your skincare routine, especially for improving fine lines and overall skin tone. However, for deeper skin issues, it's better to seek professional treatments.

Understanding Why Some People Don't See Results

Not everyone will experience immediate or dramatic results from microneedling, and patience is often necessary. The skin's healing and collagen production processes take time, meaning that results can be gradual and may require multiple sessions. It typically takes 4 to 6 sessions spaced a few weeks apart for most people to see substantial changes in skin texture, elasticity, and tone.

Another reason for limited results can be improper technique or aftercare.

Using at-home microneedling devices too frequently or with inadequate sterilization can lead to less effective outcomes or even skin issues. Similarly, using the wrong products post-treatment, such as those containing irritating ingredients, may delay healing or compromise results. Professionals can offer guidance on effective skincare products and schedules tailored to individual needs.

Finally, individual factors like age, skin type, and lifestyle impact microneedling results. Younger skin tends to heal and regenerate faster than mature skin, which may need more sessions to show improvements. Understanding that results vary based on these factors helps set realistic expectations and ensures a smoother, more effective microneedling experience.

What To Do If Microneedling Isn't Suitable For You

If microneedling is unsuitable due to skin sensitivity, medical conditions, or personal concerns, there are alternative treatments available. Chemical peels, for instance, can help improve skin texture and tone, while laser treatments may address pigmentation and deeper scarring. Non-invasive options like microdermabrasion can also offer similar benefits by gently exfoliating the skin and promoting cell turnover without the need for needles.

Another option is using topical treatments with proven skin-rejuvenating ingredients such as retinoids, vitamin C, and hyaluronic acid. These can be combined with professional facials to enhance skin texture, moisture levels, and brightness over time. Although these alternatives may not stimulate collagen production as intensely as microneedling, they can help maintain smooth, radiant skin without the associated risks.

For those seeking a less invasive approach, regular facials, good skincare habits, and sun protection play a vital role in maintaining healthy skin. Many skincare professionals offer personalized routines and product recommendations for those who can't undergo microneedling, ensuring you can still achieve and maintain glowing skin without needles.

CHAPTER NINE

FAQs On Microneedling

Can Microneedling Help With Acne Scars?

Yes, microneedling is highly effective in improving the appearance of acne scars by stimulating collagen production in the skin. When a microneedling device creates tiny, controlled punctures, the body reacts by repairing those micro-injuries, which can lead to a smoother and more even skin texture. It typically requires multiple sessions, depending on the severity of the scars, with visible improvement often noticeable after a few treatments.

The process usually involves applying a numbing cream to the skin for comfort before using the device. The tool is then rolled or stamped over the scarred area, creating micro-channels in the skin that help products like hyaluronic acid to penetrate deeper and promote healing. Treatments are spaced about four to six weeks apart to give the skin time to recover and generate collagen between sessions.

However, microneedling may not work for everyone, particularly those with very deep or ice-pick scars, which may require more intensive treatments like laser therapy or fillers.

While it improves texture and tone, microneedling is generally not a one-time fix, and results can vary based on skin type, age, and skincare regimen.

Is Microneedling Safe During Pregnancy?

Microneedling is generally not recommended during pregnancy due to the body's heightened sensitivity and immune response. Since pregnancy often causes hormonal changes that can alter skin reactions, there's an increased risk of inflammation, pigmentation, and sensitivity, which could result in unpredictable outcomes. Even though microneedling is minimally invasive, it's safer to wait until after pregnancy and breastfeeding before undergoing the procedure.

Additionally, topical numbing creams and serums commonly used in microneedling sessions may contain ingredients that aren't advised during pregnancy.

If you're considering ways to address skincare concerns during pregnancy, consult your dermatologist for gentler, safer options such as pregnancy-safe chemical peels, moisturizers, or hydrating facials.

For those who still want to maintain their skin during pregnancy, it's best to focus on a simple skincare routine with gentle products. Pregnancy-friendly options like vitamin C serums, niacinamide, and moisturizers rich in hyaluronic acid can support skin health and keep it glowing until you're ready for post-pregnancy treatments like microneedling.

How Long Before I See Results?
Results from microneedling usually begin to appear within a few weeks of the first session, although the full effect often requires multiple

treatments over several months. Many people notice an initial improvement in skin texture and firmness within two to four weeks as the skin starts healing and collagen production increases. However, the best results typically develop gradually with repeated sessions, ideally spaced four to six weeks apart.

The overall process of skin renewal from microneedling continues for up to six months post-treatment. During this time, collagen remodeling continues, which further refines the skin's appearance, smooths fine lines, and reduces hyperpigmentation. Factors like skin type, age, and aftercare can influence how soon results appear, so following a proper post-treatment skincare routine is essential for optimal outcomes.

Using gentle, hydrating skincare products, sun protection, and avoiding harsh treatments or products post-micro needling can help maintain and enhance results. Remember that microneedling is not an instant fix; patience and consistent care will yield the most noticeable improvements over time.

Are There Alternatives To Microneedling?

Yes, several alternatives can achieve similar skin benefits for those who may not be candidates for microneedling. Chemical peels, for example, use acids to exfoliate the skin deeply and encourage new skin cell turnover, which can help reduce acne scars, pigmentation, and fine lines. Lasers, like fractional CO_2 or IPL, are also effective in stimulating collagen and improving skin texture and tone, though they may require more downtime.

For those interested in collagen stimulation without needles, radiofrequency treatments can help. Radiofrequency microneedling combines heat and micro-injuries but can be performed at different intensities, so it's an excellent option for individuals with sensitive skin. Alternatively, microdermabrasion is a gentler option for superficial skin concerns and can smooth out fine lines and improve skin tone with minimal downtime.

Each of these alternatives has its pros and cons, including cost, downtime, and the results they achieve. Consulting a dermatologist or skincare specialist can help determine the best treatment based on your skin type, goals, and tolerance for downtime or discomfort.

What Should I Do If My Skin Reacts Poorly?

If you experience redness, swelling, or irritation beyond the typical post-micro needling recovery period, it's essential to care for your skin gently and avoid applying harsh products. Start with cooling the skin using clean, cold compresses, which can soothe irritation and reduce inflammation. Following up with a hydrating, fragrance-free moisturizer can also provide relief and support skin healing.

To prevent further irritation, avoid makeup, exfoliants, or any active skincare ingredients like retinoids or acids for several days post-treatment. Stick to gentle cleansers and avoid sun exposure as much as possible, as the skin is especially vulnerable to UV damage after microneedling. Using a broad-spectrum sunscreen with SPF 30 or higher is essential when you go outside to protect healing skin.

If symptoms persist or worsen, such as the development of a rash, prolonged swelling, or signs of infection, contacts a dermatologist immediately. In most cases, reactions are mild and temporary, but professional guidance can ensure safe, effective healing and prevent potential complications.

CHAPTER TEN

Cost, Accessibility, And Finding A Practitioner

Microneedling procedures can vary in cost depending on the location, expertise of the practitioner, and type of treatment. On average, professional microneedling sessions in the U.S. range from $200 to $700 per session, and most treatments require multiple sessions for optimal results.

Clinics may also offer additional treatments like serums or growth factors, which can add to the cost. While this may seem expensive, the professional equipment and medical-grade products used in clinics often provide more noticeable and longer-lasting results.

At-home microneedling devices are significantly cheaper, with basic rollers priced between $20 and $100. However, these devices often have shorter needles and may not penetrate the skin as deeply as professional-grade tools. Although they can be a more affordable option, at-home treatments require more frequent sessions and careful sterilization to avoid infection. It's important to weigh the pros and cons of at-home treatments versus professional ones, considering factors like skin type, desired results, and budget.

When choosing a microneedling practitioner, it's crucial to find a qualified professional with experience in skin treatments. Look for certified dermatologists or licensed medical aestheticians who specialize in microneedling. Ensure the clinic uses FDA-approved equipment and follows strict hygiene practices. Always check reviews, ask for before-and-after photos, and confirm that the facility follows proper sanitation protocols to reduce the risk of infection. Many clinics offer consultations to help you make an informed decision.

Average Costs Of Microneedling Procedures

The cost of microneedling treatments can vary significantly depending on the area being treated and the complexity of the procedure. On average, face treatments cost around $300 per session, while treating larger areas like the neck or body can range from $500 to $700.

Clinics typically recommend multiple sessions spaced several weeks apart to achieve the best results, so the total cost can add up over time. Additionally, advanced microneedling treatments that incorporate platelet-rich plasma (PRP) or radiofrequency (RF) technology can raise the price even higher.

For more advanced treatments like PRP microneedling, the price can range between $600 and $1,500 per session. These higher-cost treatments are often reserved for people seeking faster or more significant improvements in their skin's texture, firmness, or tone. Some clinics may offer package deals that lower the overall cost when you purchase multiple sessions upfront, so it's worth asking about discounts.

It's important to consider your budget when planning microneedling treatments, especially since results often require several sessions. Some clinics also offer financing options, allowing patients to pay for treatments in installments. Whether opting for standard microneedling or more specialized treatments, it's advisable to have a clear understanding of the total cost, including any add-ons like serums or post-care products.

At-Home Vs. Professional Treatment Costs

At-home microneedling devices are much cheaper than professional treatments, but the results can vary. Basic derma rollers with short needles (usually 0.25 to 0.5 mm) can cost anywhere from $20 to $100, making them an affordable option for those who want to improve their skin texture or fine lines. However, at-home devices typically offer milder results compared to professional treatments because they don't penetrate as deeply into the skin. Regular use of an at-home roller may also require additional skincare products, like serums, to enhance the results, which can add to the cost.

Professional microneedling treatments, on the other hand, typically use needles between 1 mm and 2.5 mm in length. These treatments are more intensive and offer deeper skin rejuvenation but come with a higher price tag, ranging from $200 to $700 per session. Professional equipment is more precise, and practitioners are trained to ensure optimal safety and hygiene, reducing the risk of complications. For individuals with more serious skin concerns, such as deep acne scars or pigmentation issues, professional microneedling may be a more effective solution, despite the higher cost.

Choosing between at-home and professional microneedling depends on your skin goals, budget, and comfort level with DIY treatments. If you're new to microneedling and seeking mild improvements, starting with an at-home roller may be a good first step.

However, if you desire more significant changes or have safety concerns, investing in professional treatments may offer better and faster results.

Tips For Finding A Qualified Microneedling Practitioner

When searching for a qualified microneedling practitioner, it's essential to prioritize safety and expertise. Look for professionals who are certified dermatologists or licensed medical aestheticians with experience in performing microneedling treatments. Check that they have specialized training in this procedure and understand how to treat different skin types and concerns. A skilled practitioner will assess your skin before recommending a treatment plan, ensuring it's tailored to your specific needs.

Ask to see before-and-after photos of previous clients, as this can give you a good idea of the results you can expect.

Additionally, check online reviews and testimonials from other clients. Personal recommendations from friends or family members who have had successful treatments can also help you find a reliable practitioner. Don't hesitate to ask your practitioner about their experience, the equipment they use, and what safety protocols they follow during the procedure.

Finally, always schedule a consultation before committing to a treatment. During the consultation, discuss your goals, ask about potential side effects, and ensure the practitioner provides clear instructions on pre- and post-treatment care. A professional practitioner should be transparent, patient, and willing to answer all your questions.

They should also be able to explain the entire procedure and outline what you can realistically expect in terms of results.

What To Look For In A Clean And Safe Facility

The cleanliness and safety of the clinic where you undergo microneedling is a critical factors in ensuring a successful and safe treatment. Make sure the facility follows strict hygiene protocols, including the use of disposable needles and sterilized equipment.

A reputable clinic will adhere to health and safety guidelines, and practitioners should always wear gloves during the procedure. You should also observe whether they disinfect treatment areas and use medical-grade products for the procedure.

When visiting a clinic for a consultation, pay attention to the overall cleanliness of the facility. The treatment rooms should be well-maintained, and all tools and machines should be stored in sterile conditions. Ask the practitioner about their sanitation practices, particularly how they clean the microneedling devices between clients. A clinic that prioritizes safety will be transparent about its hygiene standards and procedures.

It's also essential to ensure the practitioner is licensed and that the clinic is certified to perform microneedling treatments. A clean, professional environment not only reduces the risk of infection but also ensures that the procedure is performed with care and precision.

Avoid clinics that seem unorganized or fail to meet basic cleanliness standards, as this could put your health and skin at risk.

Options For Affordable Microneedling Treatments

Microneedling can be expensive, but there are several ways to make it more affordable. Many clinics offer discounts or package deals if you purchase multiple sessions upfront. These packages often provide a significant price reduction, making it easier to commit to the recommended number of treatments.

Additionally, some dermatology offices or medspas offer promotional deals during certain times of the year, such as discounts on first-time visits or seasonal specials.

Another option for more affordable microneedling treatments is to look for training schools where licensed professionals teach students. These schools often offer discounted treatments performed by supervised trainees. While the practitioner may be less experienced, the oversight of a skilled instructor ensures that the treatment is performed safely and effectively. This can be a great way to save money while still receiving professional treatment.

For those on a tight budget, at-home microneedling is the most cost-effective option. While it may take longer to see results compared to professional treatments, at-home devices are affordable and can be used frequently without ongoing costs.

You can also ask your dermatologist for product recommendations to enhance the effects of your at-home treatments, helping you achieve better results over time without spending a fortune.

Conclusion

In conclusion, microneedling is a versatile and effective cosmetic procedure that offers a range of benefits, from improving skin texture and reducing scars to stimulating collagen production and enhancing overall skin health.

The technique involves creating controlled micro-injuries in the skin, which triggers a natural healing response, encouraging the skin to regenerate and appear firmer, smoother, and more youthful.

Whether performed by a professional using an automated microneedling pen or through an at-home device, the procedure has gained popularity due to its relatively low risk, minimal downtime, and impressive results.

The effectiveness of microneedling depends on several factors, including the depth of needle penetration, frequency of sessions, and individual skin type and concerns. While most people experience minimal discomfort and temporary redness, it's essential to follow aftercare instructions to maximize benefits and prevent complications.

Applying soothing serums, staying hydrated, avoiding direct sunlight, and steering clear of harsh skincare products are all crucial post-procedure steps to ensure optimal results.

Microneedling is not without risks, however. Potential side effects include irritation, infection, and hyperpigmentation, particularly for those with sensitive or darker skin tones. For this reason, individuals considering microneedling should consult a qualified professional to determine whether the treatment is suitable for their skin type and specific goals.

Additionally, people with certain conditions, such as active acne or rosacea, may need to avoid the procedure or pursue alternative treatments.

In summary, microneedling offers a promising solution for individuals seeking non-surgical skin rejuvenation.

It combines scientific rigor with a customizable approach, making it adaptable to various skin types and needs. With proper guidance and care, microneedling can be a valuable addition to a skincare regimen, leading to healthier, rejuvenated skin and long-lasting improvements in texture and appearance.

THE END